Gynecologic Oncology Clinical Trials Review:

Landmark Studies in Uterine Cancer

Joshua P. Kesterson, MD
Rébécca Phaëton, MD

Division of Gynecologic Oncology
Department of Obstetrics and Gynecology
Penn State Milton S. Hershey Medical Center
Hershey, Pennsylvania

Note to Reader

This book is to serve as a review of gynecologic oncology and related topics for examination preparation and review purposes. It is not intended to substitute for sound clinical judgment or to guide treatment for an individual patient. Readers are encouraged to confirm the information with other sources and keep informed of ongoing studies. The authors assume no responsibility for any errors or omissions within this book.

In the *Controversies / Questions* sections of the studies detailed, editorials are often referenced. This is not to imply that all comments listed are attributable to those particular authors, but the reference is rather to serve as a source for those looking for a more detailed discussion of that particular study's controversies and critiques.

Introduction

Approximately 100,000 women will be diagnosed with a gynecologic malignancy (i.e. uterine, ovarian, cervical, vulvar, vaginal) each year in the United States [1]. The standard of care in gynecologic oncology has been established via prospective, randomized clinical trials, comparing the current standard with promising, emerging therapies. These clinical trials have in large part been designed, implemented and reported by the cooperative group, Gynecologic Oncology Group (GOG), among others. Because of these efforts, the outcomes of women with gynecologic malignancies have markedly improved over the last several decades. It is critical that the practitioner caring for these women understand the current standard of care and utilize their knowledge to develop future studies. The *Gynecologic Oncology Clinical Trials Review* is designed for ease of use and ready comprehension, with its topics divided into disease sites and chronological order, its reader-friendly format, and condensation of entire clinical trials into salient highlights, while addressing limitations, areas of controversy and the clinical impact of the trial. This *Gynecologic Oncology Clinical Trials Book* aims to serve as an indispensable resource for gynecologic oncologists, medical oncologists, and radiation oncologists, fellows and residents, as well as a study resource and reference.

Gynecologic Oncology Clinical Trials Review: Landmark Studies in Uterine Cancer represents the first installment, with subsequent releases of ovarian cancer, cervix cancer, and vulvar cancer planned.

Feedback is appreciated. (email: jkesterson@pennstatehealth.psu.edu)

Table of Contents

Endometrial Hyperplasia: Endometrial Cancer Precursor 1

  GOG 167 (Part A)): Reproducibility of the Diagnosis of Atypical Endometrial Hyperplasia: A Gynecologic Oncology Group Study 2

  GOG 167 (Part B): Concurrent Endometrial Carcinoma in Women with a Biopsy Diagnosis of Atypical Endometrial Hyperplasia 5

Early Stage Endometrial Cancer: Surgical Assessment of Disease Extent 8

  GOG 33: Surgical pathologic spread patterns of endometrial cancer. A Gynecologic Oncology Group Study 9

  GOG LAP2: Laparoscopy Compared With Laparotomy for Comprehensive Surgical Staging of Uterine Cancer: Gynecologic Oncology Group Study LAP2 11

  ASTEC: Efficacy of systematic pelvic lymphadenectomy in endometrial cancer (MRC ASTEC trial): a randomised study 14

  Panici: Systematic Pelvic Lymphadenectomy vs No Lymphadenectomy in Early-Stage Endometrial Carcinoma: Randomized Clinical Trial 18

Adjuvant Therapy for Early Stage Endometrial Cancer 21

  GOG 99: A phase III trial of surgery with or without adjunctive external pelvic radiation therapy in intermediate risk endometrial adenocarcinoma: a Gynecologic Oncology Group study 22

  PORTEC: Surgery and postoperative radiotherapy versus surgery alone for patients with stage-1 endometrial carcinoma: multicenter randomized trial 24

  PORTEC 2: Vaginal brachytherapy versus pelvic external beam radiotherapy for patients with endometrial cancer of high-intermediate risk (PORTEC-2): an open-label, non-inferiority, randomized trial 27

  Maggi: Adjuvant chemotherapy vs radiotherapy in high-risk endometrial carcinoma: results of a randomized trial 30

  JGOG 2033: Randomized phase III trial of pelvic radiotherapy versus cisplatin-based combined chemotherapy in patients with intermediate- and high-risk endometrial cancer: A Japanese Gynecologic Oncology Group study 32

Advanced / Recurrent Endometrial Cancer: Role of Chemotherapy . 35

GOG 48: A Randomized Comparison of Doxorubicin Alone Versus Doxorubicin Plus Cyclophosphamide in the Management of Advanced or Recurrent Endometrial Carcinoma: A Gynecologic Oncology Group Study 36

GOG 107: Phase III Trial of Doxorubicin With or Without Cisplatin in Advanced Endometrial Carcinoma: A Gynecologic Oncology Group Study 38

GOG 139: Randomized Phase III Trial of Standard Timed Doxorubicin Plus Cisplatin Versus Circadian Timed Doxorubicin Plus Cisplatin in Stage III and IV or Recurrent Endometrial Carcinoma: A Gynecologic Oncology Group Study 40

GOG 163: Phase III randomized trial of doxorubicin + cisplatin versus doxorubicin + 24-h paclitaxel + filgrastim in endometrial carcinoma: a Gynecologic Oncology Group study 42

GOG 177: Phase III Trial of Doxorubicin Plus Cisplatin With or Without Paclitaxel Plus Filgrastim in Advanced Endometrial Carcinoma: A Gynecologic Oncology Group Study...44

McMeekin (GOG 107, 139, 163, 177): The relationship between histology and outcome in advanced and recurrent endometrial cancer patients participating in first-line chemotherapy trials: A Gynecologic Oncology Group study 47

GOG 209: Randomized phase III noninferiority trial of first line chemotherapy for metastatic or recurrent endometrial carcinoma: A Gynecologic Oncology Group study 49

GOG 129H: Phase II Trial of the Pegylated Liposomal Doxorubicin in Previously Treated Metastatic Endometrial Cancer: A Gynecologic Oncology Group study 50

GOG 181B: Phase II trial of trastuzumab in women with advanced or recurrent HER2-positive endometrial cancer: A Gynecologic Oncology Group study..52

GOG 229E: Phase II Trial of Bevacizumab in Recurrent or Persistent Endometrial Cancer: A Gynecologic Oncology Group Study 54

Advanced Endometrial Cancer: Role of Chemotherapy, Radiation....56

GOG 122: Randomized Phase III Trial of Whole-Abdominal Irradiation Versus Doxorubicin and Cisplatin Chemotherapy in Advanced Endometrial Carcinoma: A Gynecologic Oncology Group Study..........57

GOG 184: A randomized phase III trial in advanced endometrial carcinoma of surgery and volume directed radiation followed by cisplatin and doxorubicin with or without paclitaxel: A Gynecologic Oncology Group study...60

Hormonal Therapy: The Role of Hormonal Therapy in Advanced / Recurrent Endometrial Cancer 63

GOG 81: Oral Medroxyprogesterone Acetate in the Treatment of Advanced or Recurrent Endometrial Carcinoma: A Dose-Response Study by the Gynecologic Oncology Group...64

GOG 81F: Tamoxifen in the Treatment of Advanced or Recurrent Endometrial Carcinoma: A Gynecologic Oncology Group Study.........67

GOG 121: High-Dose Megestrol Acetate in Advanced or Recurrent Endometrial Carcinoma: A Gynecologic Oncology Group Study.........69

GOG 119: Phase II study of medroxyprogesterone acetate plus tamoxifen in advanced endometrial carcinoma: a Gynecologic Oncology Group study...71

GOG 153: Phase II trial of alternating courses of megestrol acetate and tamoxifen in advanced endometrial carcinoma: a Gynecologic Oncology Group study...73

GOG 168: Phase II trial of alternating courses of megestrol acetate and tamoxifen in advanced endometrial carcinoma: a Gynecologic Oncology Group study...75

McMeekin arzoxifene: A phase II trial of arzoxifene, a selective estrogen response modulator, in patients with recurrent or advanced endometrial cancer 77

Uterine Carcinosarcoma: Chemotherapy, Radiotherapy in Endometrial Cancer 79

EORTC 55874: Phase III randomized study to evaluate the role of adjuvant pelvic radiotherapy in the treatment of uterine sarcomas stages I and II: An European Organisation for Research and Treatment of Cancer Gynaecological Cancer Group Study..80

GOG108: A Phase III Trial of Ifosfamide with or without Cisplatin in Carcinosarcoma of the Uterus: A Gynecologic Oncology Group Study 82

GOG 117: Adjuvant ifosfamide and cisplatin in patients with completely resected stage I or II carcinosarcomas (mixed mesodermal tumors) of the uterus: a Gynecologic Oncology Group study 84

GOG 150: A gynecologic oncology group randomized phase III trial of whole abdominal irradiation (WAI) vs. cisplatin-ifosfamide and mesna

(CIM) as post-surgical therapy in stage I–IV carcinosarcoma (CS) of the uterus 86

GOG 161: Phase III Trial of Ifosfamide With or Without Paclitaxel in Advanced Uterine Carcinosarcoma: A Gynecologic Oncology Group Study 89

Leiomyosarcoma (LMS): Chemotherapy, Radiotherapy in Uterine LMS 91

GOG 131C: Evaluation of paclitaxel in previously treated leiomyosarcoma of the uterus: a gynecologic oncology group study 92

GOG 131E: Phase II trial of gemcitabine as second-line chemotherapy of uterine leiomyosarcoma: a Gynecologic Oncology Group (GOG) Study 94

Hensley (unresectable LMS): Gemcitabine and Docetaxel in Patients With Unresectable Leiomyosarcoma: Results of a Phase II Trial 96

Hensley (resectable LMS): Adjuvant gemcitabine plus docetaxel for completely resected stages I-IV high grade uterine leiomyosarcoma: Results of a prospective study 98

GOG 131G: Fixed-dose rate gemcitabine plus docetaxel as first-line therapy for metastatic uterine leiomyosarcoma: A Gynecologic Oncology Group phase II trial...100

GOG 87J: Phase II evaluation of liposomal doxorubicin (Doxil) in recurrent or advanced leiomyosarcoma of the uterus: a Gynecologic oncology Group study 102

Special Topics 104

KEYNOTE-028: Safety and Antitumor Activity of Pembrolizumab in Advanced Programmed Death Ligand 1-Positive Endometrial Cancer: Results from the KEYNOTE-028 Study 105

GOG 137: Randomized Double-Blind Trial of Estrogen Replacement Therapy Versus Placebo in Stage I or II Endometrial Cancer: A Gynecologic Oncology Group Study 107

List of commonly used abbreviations

AEH   atypical endometrial hyperplasia

BSO   bilateral salpingo-oophorectomy

CR   complete response

CS   carcinosarcoma

DOD   dead of disease

doxo   doxorubicin

Dz   disease

EBRT   external beam radiation therapy

EIN   endometrial intraepithelial neoplasia

Hyst   hysterectomy

LN   lymph node

LND   lymph node dissection

LMS   leiomoysarcoma

MA   megestrol acetate

MI   myometrial invasion

MPA   medroxyprogesterone acetate

NS   non-significant

ORR   overall response rate (complete response + partial response)

PR   partial response

QOL   quality of life

RT   radiation therapy

TAH   total abdominal hysterectomy

Tx   treatment

VBT   vaginal brachytherapy

WAI   whole abdominal irradiation

WLE   wide local excision

Endometrial Hyperplasia:

Endometrial Cancer Precursor

GOG 167 (Part A)

Reproducibility of the Diagnosis of Atypical Endometrial Hyperplasia: A Gynecologic Oncology Group Study [2]

Background: The currently used classification system for endometrial hyperplasia was originally detailed by Kurman et al [3]

		Architecture	
		Simple	**Complex**
Nuclear atypia	(-)	Simple without atypia	Complex without atypia
	(+)	Simple with atypia	Complex with atypia

There is concern amongst pathologists regarding the reproducibility of these classifications

Objective: To prospectively determine the reproducibility of referring institutions' pathologic diagnosis of atypical endometrial hyperplasia (AEH).

Patients: 306 enrolled with 302 women with biopsy-confirmed diagnosis of AEH made by the referring institutions' pathologists

Enrollment criteria: Diagnosis of AEH made by referring institution's pathologist on a sample obtained by D&C, Novak curettage, Vebra aspirate or pipette endometrial biopsy with a hysterectomy performed within 12 weeks of diagnosis of AEH

Years: 1998 - 2003

Results:

Agreement with diagnosis of referring pathologist diagnosis of AEH by panel majority of 3 pathologists with expertise in gynecologic pathology: 38% of cases.

Complete (3 of 3 gynecologic pathologists) agreement with referring institution's pathologist's diagnosis of AEH in only 15% of cases.

Biopsy interpreted as carcinoma: 29% of cases

Unanimous agreement among all three pathologists for any diagnosis: 40% of cases

Conclusions: The reproducibility of referring institution's pathologist's diagnosis of AEH is only fair.

Reproducibility of classification of same cases among panel of gynecologic pathologists is only fair (kappa 0.34 – 0.43)

Diagnosis of AEH in endometrial sample associated with high frequency of adenocarcinomas and low level of reproducibility

Controversies /Questions:

A concurrent agreement by gynecologic pathologists with AEH diagnosis in 38% of cases may actually be an over-representation as all reviewing pathologist knew that the submitted specimens were initially diagnosed as AEH.

The gold standard for diagnosis is not consensus among the gynecologic pathologist panel but rather the subsequent hysterectomy specimen.

The poor reproducibility in GOG 167 was demonstrated in a subsequent study involving 1,799 women and nearly 2,500 specimens, where they reported a 49.8% agreement for atypical hyperplasia and 57.5% agreement for adenocarcinoma [4]

This poor reproducibility is also true for tumor grading [5, 6]

What is the best classification system which is biologically meaningful? Reproducible? And predictive of hysterectomy findings?

GOG 167 (Part B)

Concurrent Endometrial Carcinoma in Women with a Biopsy Diagnosis of Atypical Endometrial Hyperplasia: A Gynecologic Oncology Group Study [7]

Background: Endometrioid-type endometrial cancers develop in a continuum, with endometrial hyperplasia with atypia being a precursor lesion

Objective: Determine the prevalence of concurrent endometrial carcinoma in women with diagnosis of atypical endometrial hyperplasia (AEH)

Patients: 306 enrolled; 289 eligible with community hospital pathologic diagnosis of AEH undergoing hysterectomy within 12 weeks of initial diagnosis

Enrollment criteria: Women with community hospital pathology diagnosis of AEH who underwent subsequent hysterectomy within 12 weeks of study and had no interval treatment; hysterectomy specimens were reviewed separately from the corresponding pre-operative biopsies

Years: 1998 – 2003

Results:

Community hospital diagnosis of AEH	
Hysterectomy specimen with endometrial cancer	42.6%
Endometrial cancer extent	
Endometrium only	65%
Myoinvasive	30.9%
Outer half myometrial invasion	10.6%
High grade (2, 3)	6.5%

Conclusions: The prevalence of endometrial cancer in patients who had a community hospital diagnosis of AEH was high (42.6%)

Controversies / Questions:

The risk of concurrent endometrial cancer has implications for surgical management and appropriate referral. Recommendations by a National Institutes of Health (NIH) panel include [8]:

> "Exclusion of concurrent carcinoma is a necessary diagnostic goal of the patient newly diagnosed with AEH or EIN"

> "Consultation with a physician experienced in the management of these lesions should help the gynecologist choose the appropriate surgical procedure."

> "If hysterectomy is performed for atypical endometrial hyperplasia or endometrial intraepithelial neoplasia,

intraoperative assessment of the uterine specimen for occult carcinoma is desirable, but optional."

Should additional imaging modalities be implemented to determine if myometrial invasion is present as a means of initiating appropriate referral?

Early Stage Endometrial Cancer:

Surgical Assessment of Disease Extent

GOG 33

Surgical Pathologic Spread Patterns of Endometrial Cancer. A Gynecologic Oncology Group Study [9]

Background: Prior to this study, endometrial cancer was clinically staged

Debate as to the sequencing of RT for endometrial cancer (pre-hyst versus post-hyst)

Objective: To evaluate the surgical pathologic findings in patients with clinical stage I (confined to uterus) endometrial cancer undergoing TAH, BSO, lymphadenectomy

Patients: 621 patients with clinical stage I carcinoma of the endometrium who underwent TAH, BSO, LND and peritoneal washings

Years: 1977 - 1983

Results:

Laparotomy, peritoneal washings, pelvic and para-aortic LND, TAH, BSO (surgery aborted if LNs + for metastasis on frozen section)	
Patients with adenocarcinoma	74%
Malignant peritoneal cytology	12%
Metastasis to one or both adnexa	5%
Pelvic LN metastasis	9%
Metastasis to both pelvic and para-aortic LNs	3% (2% with metastasis to para-aortic LNs only)

Grade of tumor was correlated with frequency of nodal metastasis

Depth of invasion correlated with degree of differentiation (Table 2 in article)

Depth of invasion correlated with risk of nodal metastasis (Tables 5 & 6)

Conclusions: "This study does confirm that a significant number of patients with stage I disease can have extrauterine disease. It suggests that certain patients have significant risk of lymph node metastases and histologic evaluation of the regional lymph nodes is warranted. By applying this information to individual patients hopefully the true extent of disease can be determined, appropriate therapy applied and survival impacted."

Impact: It is hard to overstate the impact of this paper. Prompted staging for endometrial cancer change from clinical to surgical (1988 FIGO staging)

GOG LAP2

Laparoscopy Compared With Laparotomy for Comprehensive Surgical Staging of Uterine Cancer: Gynecologic Oncology Group Study LAP2 [10]

Background: In 1990s, laparoscopy was used to obtain the same goals of staging endometrial cancer traditionally done via laparotomy

Objective: To compare laparoscopy versus laparotomy for surgical staging of uterine cancer

Patients: 2,616 women with clinical stage I-IIA uterine cancer

Years: 1996 – 2005

Treatment arms:

	Laparotomy N=920	Laparoscopy N=1,696	P value
Operative time	130 min.	204 min.	
Conversion to laparotomy	n/a	26%*	
Intraoperative complications	8%	10%	0.106
Post-op. complications (≥G2)	21%	14%	<.001
Hospital stay > 2 days	94%	52%	<.0001

Ileus	7%	4%	<.004
Pelvic LNs obtained	99%	98%	0.183
Para-aortic LNs obtained	97%	94%	0.002

*Reasons for conversion: poor exposure (57%); cancer resection (16%); excessive bleeding (11%)

Conclusions: Laparoscopic surgical staging for endometrial cancer is feasible and safer than laparotomy in terms of short-term outcomes

Controversies / Questions [11]: Relatively high rate of conversion to laparotomy.

Likelihood of conversion to laparotomy increased with higher BMI and age (patients that would benefit most from not having a laparotomy).

No recurrence or survival data reported

What is the role of surgical staging in presumed early stage endometrial cancer?

Is the BMI of 28 in this study similar to that seen in women with endometrial cancer in clinical practice?

Is there a need to further discriminate between laparoscopic and robotic-assisted laparoscopic hysterectomy?

Follow-up: A Cochrane review evaluating laparoscopy versus laparotomy for the management of early stage endometrial cancer (including 3,644 women in 8 randomized controlled trials) reported similar overall and disease-free survival [12].

Laparoscopy was associated with reduced operative morbidity and shorter hospital stay.

A recent multinational randomized trial in patients undergoing surgical management of their presumed stage I uterine endometrioid adendecarcinoma demonstrated similar disease free survival between patients in the TAH group and the total laparoscopic hysterectomy group [13]

Comment: Rather impressive that 2,600 women enrolled and randomized in this trial with such discrepant initial treatment approaches

ASTEC

Efficacy of systematic pelvic lymphadenectomy in endometrial cancer (MRC ASTEC trial): a randomised study [14]

Background: Evidence is scarce regarding therapeutic benefit of lymph node dissection (LND) in regards to survival.

Pelvic LN metastases in approximately 10% of women with clinical stage I endometrial cancer.

Objective: Investigate whether pelvic LND could improve survival of women with endometrial cancer.

Years: 1998 - 2005

Patients: 1,408 women with endometrial cancer thought to be confined to the uterus

Treatment arms:

	Standard surgery group N=704	**LND group** N=704
	Hyst + BSO with No LND	**Hyst + BSO + LND**
	Hysterectomy + BSO + palpation of PALNs +/- LN sampling	Hysterectomy + BSO + pelvic LND +/- PALND
Patients divided into 1 of 3 categories	1. Low risk (IA or IB and G1 or G2) 2. Intermediate & High risk (IA or IB with G3, IC, or IIA)*	

	3. Advanced stage	
Endometrioid type	80%	79%
No nodes removed	95%	8%
Received RT	23%	23%
OS (5 year)	81%	80%
RFS (5 year)	79%	73%

* Intermediate & High risk randomized to EBRT versus no EBRT (ASTEC radiotherapy trial)

Conclusions: No evidence of a benefit for systematic lymphadenectomy for endometrial cancer in terms of RFS and OS.

Controversies / Questions [15-19]: (Also eloquently and succinctly detailed by Creasman, Mutch and Herzog [20])

The benefit of nodal dissection obscured since high risk patients were subsequently randomized and therefore half did not receive adjuvant RT

The lymphadenectomy had more high-risk features (poor histologic subtypes, grade 3 lesions, LVSI, deep myometrial invasion). These are risk factors for metastatic spread and therefore more adversely impact outcomes.

The trial may be statistically underpowered to assess the primary endpoint.

Intent-to-treat analysis despite protocol violations regarding treatment including:

1. Patients unfit for LND in the surgery study could be randomized to RT study with or without having had LND

2. Even if pre-op CT demonstrated nodal enlargement these patients were still included in study and randomized

3. 5% of the no-LND arm had LNs removed with nearly 30% of those having LN metastases

4. The LN dissection in the 'node' group may have been inadequate

As 8% in the LND group had no LNs removed and 35% of LND patients with ≤9 LNs removed

A majority of patients in surgical trial not included in the 2nd randomization (RT) but many received adjuvant therapy (EBRT, brachytherapy, or combination)

In patients with advanced disease, only 25% received aggressive adjuvant therapy with chemotherapy

Surgery was also allowed via laparoscopy

Many low risk endometrial carcinomas included

Did not assess para-aortic lymph nodes

Palpation of lymph nodes is an inaccurate predictor of disease status (GOG 33) [9]

28% of deaths not related to treatment or disease

The absolute difference in RFS increased over time in favor of Hyst + BSO with No LND group

Questions:

Are there subgroups of patients that would derive therapeutic benefit from systematic surgical staging?

Panici_Pelvic Lymphadenectomy vs No Lymphadenectomy

Systematic Pelvic Lymphadenectomy vs No Lymphadenectomy in Early-Stage Endometrial Carcinoma: Randomized Clinical Trial [21]

Background: Lymphadenectomy is important in the surgical staging of endometrial cancer.

Lymph nodes are most common site of metastasis in endometrial cancer.

Patients with metastases to lymph nodes have worse prognosis.

Lymphadenectomy may have therapeutic value [22]

Objective: To determine if the addition of systematic pelvic lymphadenectomy to hysterectomy and BSO improve overall survival and progression-free survival in patients with clinically suspected stage I endometrial cancer

Patients: 514 eligible patients with preoperative clinical stage I endometrial cancer; endometrioid or adenosquamous histology; those with well-differentiated tumors with <50% MI (on intraoperative exam) excluded

Years: 1996 – 2006

Treatment arms:

	Hysterectomy + BSO		P value
	Lymphadenectomy (pelvic LNs +/- aortic LNs) >20 LNs required	**No lymphadenectomy** (LNs removed only if >1 cm LNs noted intraoperatively)	
Pelvic LND	100%*	22%	
Lymph node metas.	13%	3%	<.001
Aortic LNs removed	26%	2%	
Stage ≥ II	26%	20%	
OR time	180 min	120 min	<.001
No adjuvant tx.	69%	65%	.07
PFS (5 year)	81%	82%	0.68
OS (5 year)	86%	90%	0.50
Post-op complications	31%	14%	<.001
Lymphedema	13%	1.6%	<.05
Lymph node metas.	13%	3%	<.001

*14% with <20 LNs removed

Conclusions: Systemic pelvic lymphadenectomy did not improve disease-free or overall survival, however it improved surgical staging.

Controversies / Questions [23, 24]:

Adjuvant therapy not standardized.

How to account for any differences between arms in regards to adjuvant therapy, based on diagnosis of metastatic disease discovered via lymphadenectomy?

What role would pre-operative imaging have in determining the need for surgical staging?

What effect does stage migration have on prior studies demonstrating survival differences in patients undergoing lymphadenectomy?

Is lymphadenectomy warranted for its prognostic and its adjuvant therapy implications?

Adjuvant Therapy for Early Stage Endometrial Cancer

GOG 99

A phase III trial of surgery with or without adjunctive external pelvic radiation therapy in intermediate risk endometrial adenocarcinoma: a Gynecologic Oncology Group study [25]

Background: Post-operative RT has been used in an attempt to decrease relapses in endometrial cancer patients

Objective: Assess the utility of post-operative RT in women with stage IB, IC and II (occult) endometrial cancer

Patients: 392 eligible women with stage IB, IC and II (1988 FIGO staging) endometrial cancer; s/p TAH, BSO, *selective* bilateral pelvic and para-aortic LND clear cell and serous types excluded

Years: 1987 – 1995

Treatment:

	No Adjuvant Treatment (NAT)	RT* EBRT 50.4 Gy	P value
Recurrence (2 yrs)	12%	3%	.007
HIR[‡] group recurrence (2 yrs)	26%	6%	
Isolated vaginal recurrence (2 yrs)	7.4%	1.6%	
OS (4 yrs)	86%	92%	0.56
Adverse events (G1-4)			

Hematologic	10%	35%	<0.001
Gastrointestinal	7%	67%	<0.001
Genitourinary	8%	30%	<0.001

*RT Borders: L4-5 interspace, mid-portion obturator foramen, 1 cm beyond lateral margins of bony pelvis

‡ HIR: moderate to poorly differentiated tumor, LVSI, and outer third myometrial invasion; >50 years old and any 2 risk factors; >70 years old and any 1 risk factor

Conclusions: Adjuvant pelvic RT reduces the risk of recurrence. Survival was not improved.

Controversies /Questions [26, 27]: Study designed on belief that risk of recurrence for intermediate risk endometrial cancer was 20 – 25%.

Lymph node counts not required for enrollment.

Half of deaths secondary to non-endometrial cancer causes.

Majority of patients in study (66%) at low risk for recurrence.

Heterogeneity of patients and risk of recurrence in the HIR group (e.g. 70 yo with superficially invasive G2 and a woman with a deeply invasive G3 tumor)

Even without addition of RT, a majority of patients did not recur.

Would vaginal brachytherapy be as effective?...PORTEC 2

What about approach of withholding post-operative RT and radiating only those patients who develop vaginal recurrence?

PORTEC

Surgery and postoperative radiotherapy versus surgery alone for patients with stage-1 endometrial carcinoma: multicentre randomised trial [28]

Background: Role of RT after TAH/BSO for early stage endometrial cancer is controversial

Objective: Compare locoregional control, overall survival and treatment-related morbidity of patients with stage I endometrial cancer treated with post-operative radiotherapy versus surgery alone

Patients: 714 patients with stage I endometrial cancer s/p TAH/BSO (*without routine LND*); Eligiblility criteria: stage I, grade 1 with ≥ 50% myometrial invasion (MI), grade 2 with any MI or grade 3 with < 50% MI

Years: 1990 – 1997

Treatment arms:

	Control	**RT**	P value
	No further treatment	Pelvic RT: 46 Gy (2 Gy/fraction)	
Locoregional recurrence (73% vaginal)	14%	4%	<.001
Distant metastases	7%	8%	

Overall survival (5 yr)*	85%	81%	.31
Adverse effects			
Late complications#	6%	25%	<.001
GI (Grade 3)	0.28%	1.7%	

*most deaths (61%) not related to endometrial cancer, i.e. cardiovascular, secondary malignancies

#Most (68%) of complications were grade 1

‡Most (73%) of recurrences restricted to vagina

Conclusions: For selected stage I patients, post-operative RT improved local control but did not translate into a survival advantage

Controversies / Questions [29, 30]: The proportion of patients who died of endometrial cancer-related causes was higher in RT group (9% versus 6%, p value 0.37)

No staging requirement (unlike GOG 99)

Salvage treatment after vaginal relapse in the control arm (no RT) often successful

Although 23 of 51 patients with locoregional recurrence died, but only 7 due to their recurrence (2-year survival after vaginal recurrence: 79%)

Pathology review resulted in significantly more tumors classified as grade 1.

What is role of universal prophylactic radiation to prevent a recurrence that only a minority of patients will develop? And which only a minority of those patients will ultimately die of?

In the absence of survival benefit, shouldn't postoperative radiotherapy reduce morbidity to be of value?

Considering that a majority of locoregional recurrences are vaginal, would vaginal brachytherapy be as effective as pelvic RT? ...PORTEC2

PORTEC 2

Vaginal brachytherapy versus pelvic external beam radiotherapy for patients with endometrial cancer of high-intermediate risk (PORTEC-2): an open-label, non-inferiority, randomized trial [31]

Background: GOG 99 and PORTEC1 compared pelvic EBRT versus no adjuvant therapy for early stage endometrial cancer and showed a decreased rate of local-regional recurrence with RT.

In PORTEC, adverse effects (predominantly GI) in 26% of patients receiving EBRT

Retrospective studies have reported vaginal brachytherapy (VBT) as being effective in prevention of vaginal recurrence.

In PORTEC, adverse effects in 26% of patients receiving EBRT (predominantly GI)

Objective: Investigate if VBT would be equally effective as pelvic EBRT in prevention of vaginal recurrence, with fewer treatment related side effects and improved quality of life

Patients: 427 women with TAH/BSO (no routine LND); eligible if: 1) >60 years old with stage IC (G1 or G2) or stage IB (G3); & 2) stage IIA, any age (except G3 with >50% myometrial invasion)

Years: 2002 – 2006

Treatment arms:

	EBRT (n=214)	**VBT** (n=213)	P value
	46 Gy in 23 fractions	21 Gy in 3 fractions (HDR) or 30 Gy (LDR) or 28 Gy (MDR)	
Vaginal recurrences (45 months)	1.6% (n=4)	1.8% (n=3)	0.74
Pelvic recurrences*	0.5%	3.8%	.02
Distant metastases	5.7%	8.3%	.46
RFS (5 years)	78%	83%	0.74
OS	80%	85%	0.57
Adverse events			
Early GI toxicity (G1-G2)‡	54%	13%	<.05

*most patients with pelvic recurrence had simultaneous distant metastases

‡Difference between arms decreased with time and lost statistical significance at 24 m.

Conclusions: VBT effective in preventing vaginal recurrences in early stage endometrial cancer.

Controversies / Questions [32]:

No lymphadenectomy required for study enrollment

Tumor grading showed poor reproducibility

On *post hoc* pathology review: 14% of patients reclassified (as either high risk or low risk and thus in retrospect ineligible).

Higher rate of distant metastasis and lower survival in those determined to be high risk or advanced stage on pathologic reclassification (versus true high-intermediate risk)

Isolated vaginal recurrences can be salvaged in radiation naïve women.

RT in this setting demonstrated no survival advantage

Was the margin of non-inferiority too wide?

Follow-up:

In a QOL follow up at 2 years, those patients who received EBRT had higher levels of diarrhea and bowel symptoms resulting in limitations in daily activities and decreased social functioning [33]

Maggi

Adjuvant chemotherapy vs radiotherapy in high-risk endometrial carcinoma: results of a randomized trial [34]

Background: PORTEC and GOG 99 demonstrated that pelvic RT improved local control, but not overall survival in women with low risk and intermediate risk endometrial cancer

Local RT does not prevent distant metastases

Objective: To assess whether adjuvant chemotherapy improves PFS and OS versus standard pelvic RT for patients with high-risk endometrial cancer

Patients: 491 referred; 345 eligible with stage endometrioid adenocarcinoma stage IC grade 3; IIA-B grade 3 with deep myometrial invasion (≥50%) or stage III disease; TAH/BSO +/- LND; (2/3rds of pts Stage III)

Years: 1990 – 1997

Treatment arms:

	RT* (n=166)	**Chemotherapy** (n=174)	P value
	EBRT 45-50 Gy (over 5-7 weeks)	Cyclophosphamide 600 mg/m^2 & Adriamycin 45 mg/m^2 & Cisplatin 50 mg/m^2	
		Q28 days x 5 cycles	

Completed tx	88%	75%	
PFS (3 year)	69%	68%	NS
OS (3 year)	78%	76%	NS
Adverse effects	Bowel obstruction (5) Radiation proctitis (6)	Neutropenia (G3&4) 35% Anemia (G2&3) 33%	

*RT borders: upper=L5, lower=lower limit of ischial tuberosity; lateral=lateral and common iliac lymph nodes

Conclusions: No improvement in PFS and OS in patients treated with adjuvant chemotherapy vesus adjuvant radiotherapy

Controversies / Questions: Patients with a rather heterogenous risk profile (i.e. stage IC to stage III)

Would RT + chemotherapy in sequence or in series be more effective than either independently in the adjuvant setting?

Cyclophosphamide not a standard agent in phase III GOG endometrial trials

JGOG 2033

Randomized phase III trial of pelvic radiotherapy versus cisplatin-based combined chemotherapy in patients with intermediate- and high-risk endometrial cancer: A Japanese Gynecologic Oncology Group study [35]

Background: A need to determine the optimal adjuvant treatment to decrease recurrence and improve OS in patients with early stage endometrial cancer

Objective: Compare adjuvant pelvic RT versus platinum-based chemotherapy for patients with stage IC to IIIC endometrial cancer in regards to PFS and OS

Patients: 385 patients with IC – IIIC endometrial cancer with >50% myometrial invasion, <75 years old s/p TAH, BSO, LND; majority (61%) stage IC

Years: 1994 – 2000

Treatment arms:

	Pelvic RT	Chemotherapy	P value
	45-50 Gy	Cyclophos 333 mg/m² & Doxorubicin 40 mg/m² & Cisplatin 50 mg/m²	
		Q 4 wks x ≥3 cycles	

Recurrences	15.5%	17.2%	NS
Pelvis/vagina	6.7%	7.3%	NS
Extra-pelvic	13.5%	16.1%	NS
PFS (5 yrs)	83.5%	81.8%	0.726
OS (5 yrs)	85.3%	86.7%	0.268
High-intermediate risk (HIR)*			
PFS (5 yrs)	66.2%	83.8%	0.024
OS (5 yrs)	73.6%	89.7%	0.006

*HIR: stage IC >70 yrs old or G3; stage II or IIIA (+cytology) >50% myometrial invasion

Conclusions: No difference in survival between adjuvant chemotherapy & adjuvant RT.

Chemotherapy improved PFS and OS in HIR patients.

Controversies / Questions:

In patients receiving RT, 19% of deaths secondary to non-endometrial cancer causes (versus 50% in GOG 99)

Contrast the 'high to intermediate risk' in JGOG 2033 to 'high intermediate risk' of GOG99:

JGOG 2033	GOG99
(1) Stage IC in patients >70 y.o. or with G3 endometrioid adenocarcinoma	(1) Moderate to poorly differentiated tumor, presence of LVSI and outer third MI
(2) Stage II or IIIA (positive cytology)	(2) Age ≥50 with any two risk factors listed above
	(3) Age ≥70 with any risk factors listed above

Is this patient population representative of most patients with endometrial cancer (e.g. 18% premenopausal, a majority of patients with no co-morbidities, a majority underwent an 'extended' or 'radical' hysterectomy

Advanced / Recurrent Endometrial Cancer:

Role of Chemotherapy

GOG 48

A Randomized Comparison of Doxorubicin Alone Versus Doxorubicin Plus Cyclophosphamide in the Management of Advanced or Recurrent Endometrial Carcinoma: A Gynecologic Oncology Group Study [36]

Background:

Lack of properly conducted studies on the use of chemotherapy in advanced endometrial cancer

Phase II trials showed activity of doxorubicin and doxorubicin + cyclophosphamide combination in similar patient population

Objective: Determine if doxorubicin and/or the combination of doxorubicin + cyclophosphmide have activity in advanced or recurrent endometrial cancer?

Patients: 387 enrolled; 300 with measurable disease and 276 assessable for response advanced or recurrent endometrial cancer; chemotherapy naïve

Years: 1979-1984

Treatment arms:

	Doxo 60 mg/m² IV	**Doxo** 60 mg/m² IV & **Cyclo** 500 mg/m² IV	P value
		Q21 days x 8 cycles	
Response rate			
Complete	5%	13%	NS
Partial	17%	17%	NS
Stable disease	55%	52%	
PFS	3.2 months	3.9 months	NS
Median survival	6.7 months	7.3 months	0.48*
Adverse effects		"more frequent and severe myelosuppression and gastrointestinal toxicity"	

*Pooled estimate when adjusting for grade, presence of abdominal metastases, performance status

Conclusion: Combination of doxorubicin + cyclophosphamide not superior to doxorubicin alone

Impact: Single agent Doxorubicin the control arm in GOG 107

GOG 107

Phase III Trial of Doxorubicin With or Without Cisplatin in Advanced Endometrial Carcinoma: A Gynecologic Oncology Group Study [37]

Background:

Outcomes for those with advanced or recurrent endometrial cancer are poor.

Doxorubicin and cisplatin with activity in endometrial cancer in phase II studies.

Objective: Determine if the combination of doxorubicin + cisplatin superior to doxorubicin alone

Patients: 281 women with Stage III, IV, or recurrent endometrial carcinoma; chemotherapy-naïve

Years: 1988 - 1992

Treatment arms:

	Doxo‡ + Cisp	Doxo	P value
	Doxorubicin 60 mg/m^2 & Cisplatin 50 mg/m^2	Doxorubicin 60 mg/m^2	
	Q 3 weeks		
Response rate	42%	25%	.004

	CR	19%	8%	
	PR	23%	17%	
PFS		5.7 months	3.8 months	0.014*
OS		9.0 months	9.2 months	NS
Adverse events (≥G3)				
	Leukopenia	62%	40%	
	Thrombocytopenia	14%	2%	
	Anemia	22%	4%	
	Nausea/vomiting	13%	3%	

*adjusted for initial performance status ‡max. doxo dose allowed 500 mg/m^2

Conclusions: The combination of doxorubicin + cisplatin is superior to single agent doxorubicin in terms of response rate and PFS in patients with advanced or recurrent endometrial cancer.

Controversies / Questions:

The improved efficacy of the doublet therapy did not translate to an improved overall survival.

The improved efficacy of the doublet therapy comes at the expense of increased toxicity.

Should carboplatin be substituted for cisplatin?

Impact: Doxorubicin + cisplatin became the control arm in GOG 163 [38]

GOG 139

Randomized Phase III Trial of Standard Timed Doxorubicin Plus Cisplatin Versus Circadian Timed Doxorubicin Plus Cisplatin in Stage III and IV or Recurrent Endometrial Carcinoma: A Gynecologic Oncology Group Study [39]

Background: Platinum combination chemotherapy more effective than single agent chemotherapy.

Timing of administration of doxorubicin and cisplatin may impact response and toxicity.

Objective: To determine if circadian-timed (CT) doxorubicin + cisplatin results in improved responses versus standard-timed (ST) doxorubicin + cisplatin

Patients: 342 patients with stage III, IV or recurrent endometrial cancer; measurable disease; chemotherapy naive

Years: 1993-1996

Treatment arms:

	Standard-timed	Circadian-timed	P value
	Doxorubicin* 60 mg/m^2 IV *anytime* followed by **Cisplatin** 60 mg/m^2	**Doxorubicin*** 60 mg/m^2 IV at 6 AM **Cisplatin** 60 mg/m^2 at 6 PM	
	Q 3 weeks x 8 cycles		

RR (CR +PR)	46%	49%	
Complete	15%	17%	
Partial	31%	32%	
PFS	6.5 months	5.9 months	0.31
OS	11.2 months	13.2 months	0.21
Adverse events (≥3)			
Leukopenia	75%	64%	0.01
Nausea/emesis	10%	16%	>.05
Cardiac	4%	5%	>.05

* maximum doxorubicin dose: 420 mg/m^2

Conclusion: Circadian-timed doxorubicin + cisplatin did not result in improved response, PFS, OS versus standard-timed doxorubicin + cisplatin

Impact: "the GOG does not plan additional trials of CT chemotherapy in endometrial cancer." [39]

GOG 163

Phase III randomized trial of doxorubicin + cisplatin versus doxorubicin + 24-h paclitaxel + filgrastim in endometrial carcinoma: a Gynecologic Oncology Group study [38]

Background: Outcomes for those with advanced or recurrent endometrial cancer are poor.

GOG 107 demonstrated the superiority of doxorubicin + cisplatin over doxorubicin

Objective: Is the combination of doxorubicin + paclitaxel superior to doxorubicin + cisplatin?

Patients: Of 328 enrolled, 317 eligible with Stage III, IV, or recurrent endometrial carcinoma; chemotherapy-naïve; measurable disease

Years: 1996 - 2005

Treatment arms:

	Doxo + Cisp	**Doxo**	P value
	Doxorubicin 60 mg/m^2 Cisplatin 50 mg/m^2	Doxorubicin 60 mg/m^2 Paclitaxel 150 mg/m^2 Filgrastim Days 3-12	
	Q 3wks x 7 cycles		
Response rate	40%	43%	NS

PFS	7.2 months	6 months	NS
OS	12.6 months	13.6 months	NS
Adverse events			
Granulocytopenia (G4)	54%	50%	
Thrombocytopenia (G4)	1%	1%	
Anemia (≥G3)	8%	6%	
GI (Nausea/emesis)(≥G3)	16%	12%	

Conclusions: Substituting paclitaxel for cisplatin in combination with doxorubicin did not positively impact response rate, PFS, OS

Controversies / Questions: Paclitaxel regimen required use of filgrastim

After study design, new studies came out supporting 3-hour paclitaxel infusion

GOG 177

Phase III Trial of Doxorubicin Plus Cisplatin With or Without Paclitaxel Plus Filgrastim in Advanced Endometrial Carcinoma: A Gynecologic Oncology Group Study [40]

Background:

GOG 107 established cisplatin + doxorubicin as active regimen in advanced endometrial cancer (PFS 5.7 months)

GOG 163 demonstrated that doxorubicin + paclitaxel not superior to cisplatin + doxorubicin

Objective: Determine if the combination of doxorubicin + cisplatin + paclitaxel (TAP) is superior to cisplatin + doxorubicin (AP) in women with advanced or recurrent EC

Patients: 263 women with Stage III, Stage IV, or recurrent endometrial cancer; chemotherapy-naïve

Years: 1998 –2000

Treatment arms:

	TAP (with filgastim)	**AP**	P value
Day 1	**Doxorubicin** 45mg/m^2 **Cisplatin** 50 mg/m^2	**Doxorubicin** 60mg/m^2 **Cisplatin** 50 mg/m^2	
Day 2	**Paclitaxel** 160 mg/m^2		

	Q 3 wks x 7 cycles		
Response rate	57%	34%	<.001
Complete response	22%	7%	
PFS	8.3 months	5.3 months	<.01
OS	15.3 months	12.3 months	0.037
Adverse events			
Deaths (#)	5	0	
Neutropenia (G4)	36%	50%	
Neutropenic fever	3%	2%	
Thrombocytopenia (≥G3)	22%	3%	
Peripheral neuropathy (≥G3)	12%	1%	

Conclusions: The three drug regimen of TAP is superior to two drug regimen of AP in terms of RR, PFS, OS.

Controversies / Questions:

Does the statistically significant, but small, improvement in RR, PFS, OS with TAP warrant the additional toxicity?

Would OS in AP arm be improved if more patients received paclitaxel as first salvage therapy for persistent and/or recurrent disease?

The TAP regimen required growth factor support.

Will the toxicity associated with TAP allow for its widespread acceptance?

Impact: TAP became the control arm in GOG 209 comparing TAP to carboplatin+paclitaxel.

McMeekin (GOG 107, 139, 163, 177)

The relationship between histology and outcome in advanced and recurrent endometrial cancer patients participating in first-line chemotherapy trials: A Gynecologic Oncology Group study [41]

Background: Reports of serous and clear cell histologic subtypes having different outcome than endometrioid histology

Objective: Explore association between serous and clear cell tumors and outcomes in patients with advanced or recurrent endometrial cancer treated with chemotherapy in four GOG trials

Patients: 1203 patients with advanced / recurrent endometrial cancer (serous (18%) and clear cell (4%))

Results:

	RR	PFS	OS
Endometrioid	44%	6.4 months	12.8 months
Serous	44%	6.3 months	11.1 months*
Clear cell	32%	3.2 months*	7.9 months*

*P <0.05 when compared to all other histologies

Lower odds of response if: Black, poor performance status, and prior RT

Conclusions: Similar response rate across histologies

Poorer PFS and OS in clear cell compared to other cell typs

<u>Controversies / Questions</u>: While clear cell carcinomas appeared to do worse, the histologic subtype is such a small fraction (4%)

Overall, outcomes are poor for those with advanced or recurrent endometrial cancer treated with chemotherapy, highlighting need for novel targeted agents

GOG 209 (ABSTRACT)

Randomized phase III noninferiority trial of first line chemotherapy for metastatic or recurrent endometrial carcinoma: A Gynecologic Oncology Group study

Objective: To determine if combination of carboplatin and paclitaxel (TC) is inferior to combination of doxorubicin, cisplatin, and paclitaxel (TAP) chemotherapy with regard to survival

Patients: 1,312 patients

Years: 2003 - 2009

Treatment arms:

TC	TAP
Paclitaxel 175 mg/m^2	**Doxorubicin** 45mg/m^2
Carboplatin AUC 6	**Cisplatin** 50mg/m^2
	Paclitaxel 160 mg/m^2
Q21 days x 7	

Conclusion: TC is not interior to TAP with regards to PFS and OS (based on interim analysis results)

GOG 129H

Phase II Trial of the Pegylated Liposomal Doxorubicin in Previously Treated Metastatic Endometrial Cancer: A Gynecologic Oncology Group Study [42]

Background: Doxorubicin has activity in endometrial cancer. Pegylated liposomal doxorubicin (PLD) has different pharmacology and toxicity versus doxorubicin.

Objective: To determine the activity and toxicity of PLD in patients with persistent or recurrent endometrial cancer.

Patients: 42 patients with advanced or recurrent endometrial cancer; measurable disease; ≤1 prior cytotoxic regimen

Years: 1997 - 1998

Treatment:

	PLD 50 mg/m^2 IV Q 4 weeks
Median no. of cycles	2.5 (range: 1 – 14)
Partial response rate	10% (duration of responses: 1.1, 2.1, 3.3, 5.4 months)
Stable disease rate	29%
O.S.	8.2 months
Adverse effects	
Mucositis (≥G3)	2%

Dermatologic (≥G3)	9%
Neutropenia (≥G3)	16%
Cardiovascular (G1-4)	9% (3 of 4 patients with a decrease in ejection fraction had received prior doxorubicin)

Conclusions: PLD has limited activity in this population, but favorable side-effect profile

Controversies / Questions: Considering the favorable side-effect profile and modest activity, should PLD be combined with an additional cytotoxic agent for patients with recurrent or metastatic endometrial cancer?

GOG 181B

Phase II trial of trastuzumab in women with advanced or recurrent HER2-positive endometrial cancer: A Gynecologic Oncology Group study [43]

Background: Trastuzumab, anti-HER2 monoclonal antibody, has been effective in treatment of women with HER2-positive breast cancer.

Endometrial cancer can overexpress HER2.

Purpose: Evaluate the efficacy of trastuzumab in advanced or recurrent HER2-positive endometrial cancer

Years: 2000 - 2002, 2004 - 2007

Patients: 33 patients with stage III, IV or recurrent HER2-positive endometrial cancer; measurable disease

Treatment:

	Trastuzumab 4mg/kg week 1, then 2mg/kg weekly (until progression)	
Median # of cycles	2	
Stable Dz.	36%	
Progressive Dz.	55%	
	Period A (IHC +)	Period B (HER2 ampl.)
PFS	1.84 months	1.81 months

OS	7.85 months	6.80 months

Conclusions: Single agent trastuzumab did not demonstrate activity against endometrial cancer with HER2 overexpression or HER2 amplification

Controversies / Questions:

Originally "HER2 positive" was based on IHC ("Period A") but was changed when first 23 IHC HER2-positive tumors did not have a response therefore the "HER2 positive" then required HER2 amplification ("Period B")

Trial closed early secondary to poor accrual

Does response differ by histologic type?

Would trastuzumab be more effective in combination with other chemotherapies?

GOG 229E

Phase II Trial of Bevacizumab in Recurrent or Persistent Endometrial Cancer: A Gynecologic Oncology Group Study [44]

Background: Bevacizumab has been shown to induce responses in ovarian and cervical cancer.

Objective: Evaluate activity and tolerability of bevacizumab in recurrent or persistent endometrial cancer

Patients: 52 patients with recurrent or persistent endometrial cancer; measurable disease; one or two prior cytotoxic regimens

Years: 2006 – 2007

Treatment:

	Bevacizumab 15 mg/kg IV Q 21 days
RR (CR + PR)	13.5%
Complete response (CR)	2%
Partial response (PR)	11.5%
PFS	4.17 months
OS	10.55 months
Adverse effects	
Hemorrhage (≥G3)	4%
Hypertension (≥G3)	8%

VTE (≥G3)	4%
Proteinuria (≥G3)	4%
GI perforation or fistulae	0%

Conclusion: Bevacizumab is well tolerated and active based on PFS at 6 months in recurrent or persistent endometrial cancer

Controversies / Questions: High circulating VEGF-A levels associated with poor outcomes (i.e. lack of tumor response and death)

Note to reader: This article's discussion has a well-written synopsis of the current state of single agent targeted agents in endometrial cancer

Advanced Endometrial Cancer:

Role of Chemotherapy, Radiation

GOG 122

Randomized Phase III Trial of Whole-Abdominal Irradiation Versus Doxorubicin and Cisplatin Chemotherapy in Advanced Endometrial Carcinoma: A Gynecologic Oncology Group Study [45]

Background: Relapse of endometrial cancer in abdomen has prompted use of whole abdominal irradiation (WAI).

Reported long-term survival for stage III/IV patients treated with WAI [46]

Objective: Compare WAI versus doxorubicin + cisplatin in women with stage III/IV endometrial cancer

Patients: 422 enrolled; 388 eligible women with stage III or IV endometrial; post-operative residual disease ≤ 2 cm

Years: 1992-2000

Treatment arms:

	TAH/BSO/staging (no single site of residual disease >2cm)		
	WAI	Doxo + Cis	P value
	30 Gy in 20 fractions AP/PA with boost to pelvis +/- extended field	Doxorubicin 60 mg/m^2 Cisplatin 50 mg/m^2 Q 3 weeks x 8	

		cycles	
Completed tx.	84%	63%	
Alive NED (5 year)	38%	50%	<0.05
Alive (5 year)	42%	55%	<0.05
Adverse effects			
Tx-related deaths	5 patients	8 patients	
Heme (≥G3)	14%	88%	
GI (≥G3)	13%	20%	
Received subsequent tx.	35%	45%	

<u>Conclusions</u>: doxorubicin + cisplatin resulted in improved PFS and OS in women with advanced endometrial cancer when compared to whole abdominal radiation.

<u>Controversies / Questions</u>: Despite an increased percentage of patients with poor prognostic factors in the chemotherapy arm, including metastatic aortic nodes, intra-abdominal disease, these patients had an improved 5-year PFS. This improved outcome came at the expense of increased toxicity.

Chemotherapy was scheduled for 8 cycles, of which only 63% completed. Reasons for discontinuing chemotherapy: toxicity (17%), progression (9%), patient refusal (7%)

What about a combination of RT + chemotherapy?...

Impact: This trial is often cited as the impetus for the paradigm shift in the treatment of advanced endometrial cancer toward chemotherapy.

GOG 184

A randomized phase III trial in advanced endometrial carcinoma of surgery and volume directed radiation followed by cisplatin and doxorubicin with or without paclitaxel: A Gynecologic Oncology Group study [47]

Background: GOG 107 demonstrated improved response rate with combination of doxorubicin + cisplatin over doxorubicin

GOG 122 compared WAI versus Doxorubicin + Cisplatin

Paclitaxel demonstrated responses in advanced/recurrent endometrial cancer

A combination of chemotherapy + radiation may reduce recurrence rates

Objective: Compare PFS and toxicity between doxorubicin + cisplatin (D + C) with or without paclitaxel in patients with stage III or IV endometrial cancer (≤ 2cm residual disease) after surgery and tumor directed RT

Patients: 659 enrolled; 552 eligible with stage III or IV endometrial cancer with disease <2cm after surgery with disease limited to abdomen (initially in study) or pelvis

Years: 2000-2004

Treatment arms:

	TAH/BSO +/- LND	
	RT*: tumor volume directed pelvis RT (50.4 Gy) +/- para-aortic +/- vaginal boost RT	
	If no evidence of persistent disease …	
	D + C	**D + C + T**
Day 1	**Doxorubicin** 45 mg/m^2 IV **Cisplatin** 50 mg/m^2 IV	**Doxorubicin** 45 mg/m^2 IV **Cisplatin** 50 mg/m^2 IV
Day 2		**Paclitaxel** 160 mg/m^2 IV
	Q 3 weeks x 6	
Received 6 cycles	83%	78%
RFS (3 yrs)	62%	64%
Adverse events (≥ G3)		
Neutropenia[‡]	47%	68%
Thrombocytopenia[‡]	10%	24%
Neuropathy[‡]	2%	9%

*Pelvic RT boundaries: L5/S1 interspace, obturator foramen, 1.5 cm beyond lateral margins of true pelvis

[‡] $P<0.01$ (based on maximum grade reported for all 6 cycles)

Conclusions: The addition of paclitaxel to doxorubicin + cisplatin, following adjuvant RT for stage III and IV endometrial cancer patients, did not improve PFS and was associated with more toxicity

Controversies/Questions: Results of GOG 122 came out during this trial, demonstrating superiority of chemotherapy over WAI thus initial eligibility requirements of GOG184 was amended such that patients with disease outside of pelvis (i.e. stage IV) except positive para-aortic LNs were not eligible

552 (84%) of 659 patients enrolled ultimately initiated chemotherapy

All histologies eligible (18% of patients with clear cell or serous histology)

In subgroup analysis, the D + C + T regimen was associated with a decreased risk of recurrence and deaths in those with macroscopic residual disease after surgery

Impact: The results of GOG 122, demonstrating superiority of chemotherapy over radiation in the same subset of patients came out after this trial was opened thus limiting its impact. Cisplatin + doxorubicin + paclitaxel had already demonstrated superiority over cisplatin + doxorubicin in GOG 177.

Hormonal Therapy:

The Role of Hormonal Therapy in Advanced / Recurrent Endometrial Cancer

GOG 81

Oral Medroxyprogesterone Acetate in the Treatment of Advanced or Recurrent Endometrial Carcinoma: A Dose-Response Study by the Gynecologic Oncology Group [48]

Background: Endometrial cancer is hormonally driven, responsive

Objective: Determine if a higher dose of oral progestin (medroxyprogesterone acetate (MPA)) results in an improved response rate in endometrial cancer

Patients: 299 eligible patients with advanced (stage III or IV) or recurrent endometrial cancer; measurable disease; chemotherapy naïve

Years: 1985 – 1989

Treatment arms:

	Low dose	**High dose**
	MPA **200 mg** PO QD	MPA **1000 mg** PO QD
Response rate (CR + PR)	25%	16%
Complete response (CR)	17%	9%
Partial response (PR)	8%	6%
PFS	3.2 months	2.5 months
OS	11.1 months	7.0 months

Adverse events		
Thrombophlebitis (G1-4)	5% (≥G3=2%)	4% (≥G3=2%)
Response rate varied with tumor differentiation:		
Grade	**Response rate**	P value
1	37%	<0.001
2	23%	
3	9%	
Response rate varied with receptor status:		
Receptor status	**Response rate**	P value
ER +	26%	0.005
ER -	7%	
PR +	37%	<0.001
PR -	8%	

Conclusions:

The use of MPA 200 mg/day is a reasonable approach for initial systemic treatment for advanced or recurrent endometrial cancer, especially those with well differentiated tumors and/or receptor positive

Progestin therapy is well tolerated.

Controversies / Questions: The standard initial treatment for advanced and/or recurrent endometrial cancer is cytotoxic chemotherapy.

There are no head to head comparisons of hormonal therapy versus cytotoxic chemotherapy in endometrial cancer.

16% of patients in study with serous or clear cell histology

Are there other more effective hormonal agents or combination of agents?

GOG 81F

Tamoxifen in the Treatment of Advanced or Recurrent Endometrial Carcinoma: A Gynecologic Oncology Group Study [49]

Background: Endometrial cancer is hormonally susceptible.

Objective: To determine if tamoxifen is active in advanced or recurrent endometrial cancer

Patients: 68 women with advanced or recurrent endometrial cancer; chemotherapy naïve; measurable disease

Years: 1987 – 1991

Results:

Treatment:	**Tamoxifen 20mg PO BID**
Complete response (CR)	4%
Partial response (PR)	6%
PFS	1.9 months
OS	8.8 months (31 months if fully active, i.e. performance status=0)
Adverse effects	
GI (primarily N/V)	6%
Anemia	3%

Conclusions: Tamoxifen demonstrated only modest activity in advanced / recurrent endometrial cancer.

Controversies / Questions: Responses occurred more often with well differentiated tumors (23% of G1 tumors responded versus 3% of G3)

15% of patients with serous or clear cell cancer. Would response rates be more impressive if only endometrioid type tumors were eligible for study inclusion?

Impact: "The GOG has no plans to explore further the use of tamoxifen as a single agent in endometrial carcinoma."

GOG 121

High-Dose Megestrol Acetate in Advanced or Recurrent Endometrial Carcinoma: A Gynecologic Oncology Group Study [50]

Background: GOG 81 demonstrated no improvement in response rate with higher dose of medroxyprogesterone acetate (MPA)

Serum progestin levels equivalent with MPA 1000 mg/day and megestrol acetate (MA) 160 mg/day

Objective: Assess the efficacy of MA 800 mg/day in patients with recurrent or advanced endometrial cancer

Patients: 58 women with recurrent or advanced endometrial cancer; measurable disease; no prior cytotoxic or hormonal therapy

Years: 1991 – 1992

Results:

	MA 800 mg PO QD
Complete response	11%*
Partial response	13%*
Stable disease	22%
PFS	2.5 months
OS	7.6 months
Adverse effects (G1-4)	
Weight gain	26%

Pulmonary embolism	5%
Response rate greater for GI or G2 tumors (37%) versus G3 lesions (8%)	

*median duration of response among responders =8.9 months (range: 6.5-27 months)

Conclusions: High dose MA is active in recurrent / advanced endometrial cancer (but not moreso than standard dose progetins in historical controls).

Controversies / Questions: 24% of patients in study with serous cancer. 7% response rate with serous cancer versus 33% with endometrioid histology

GOG 119

Phase II study of medroxyprogesterone acetate plus tamoxifen in advanced endometrial carcinoma: a Gynecologic Oncology Group study [51]

Background: Progestational agents and tamoxifen have demonstrated responses in endometrial cancer.

Tamoxifen has been shown to increase progesterone receptors in endometrial cancer cells.

Objective: Evaluate the response and toxicity of daily tamoxifen with intermittent weekly medroxyprogesterone acetate (MPA)

Patients: 58 evaluable recurrent or metastatic endometrial cancer patients; measurable disease; no prior cytotoxic or hormonal therapy

Years: 1991-1996

Treatment:

	Tamoxifen 20 mg PO BID + **MPA** 100 mg PO BID (on alternating (even numbered) weeks)
Response rate	
Complete response	10%
Partial response	22%
No response	67%
PFS	3 months

OS	13 months
Adverse events (G1-4)	
Thromboembolism	7%
Weight gain	35%

Conclusions: The combination of tamoxifen with intermittent weekly MPA is an active regimen for advanced or recurrent endometrial cancer.

GOG 153

Phase II trial of alternating courses of megestrol acetate and tamoxifen in advanced endometrial carcinoma: a Gynecologic Oncology Group study [52]

Background: Endometrial cancer is a hormonally sensitive neoplasm.

Tamoxifen has been shown to increase the expression of progesterone receptors.

Objective: To estimate the response and toxicity associated with alternating megesterol acetate and tamoxifen citrate in women with endometrial cancer

Patients: 56 women with recurrent or advanced endometrial cancer; no prior cytotoxic or hormonal therapy; measurable disease

Years: 1994 - 1995

Treatment:

	Megesterol acetate 80mg PO BID x 3 wks followed by **Tamoxifen** 20mg PO BID x 3 weeks (alternating)
Complete response	21%
Partial response	5%
PFS	2.7 months
OS	14 months

Adverse effects	
Weight gain	21%
Thromboembolism	9%

Note: in over half of responders, response duration exceeded 20 months

Conclusions: A regimen of alternating megesterol acetate and tamoxifen is active in recurrent and advanced endometrial cancer and may result in a prolonged response in some patients.

GOG 168

A Phase II Trial of Anastrozole in Advanced Recurrent or Persistent Endometrial Carcinoma: A Gynecologic Oncology Group Study [53]

Background: Endometrial cancers hormonally driven and responsive

Objective: Evaluate the efficacy and toxicity of anastrozole in recurrent or persistent endometrial cancer

Patients: 23 patients with advanced or recurrent endometrial cancer not curable with either surgery or radiation; measurable disease

Years: 1997 - 1998

Treatment:

	Anastrozole 1 mg/day PO
Duration of therapy	0.4 – 168 weeks (median: 4 weeks)
Partial response	9% (2 patients)
Stable disease	9% (2 patients)
PFS (median)	1 month
OS (median)	6 months
Adverse events	1 patient with VTE; 2 patients with edema (G1)

Conclusions:

"anastrozole demonstrated minimal activity in a group of women with advanced or recurrent endometrial cancer, most of whom had poorly differentiated tumors. The role of anastrozole in well-differentiated hormone-receptor-positive or hormone-sensitive endometrial carcinoma is not resolved by the present study."

Controversies / Questions:

Receptor status was not required for study entry. (Response to hormonal therapy correlates with receptor status [50, 54])

6 of 23 patients with serous or clear cell histology

McMeekin arzoxifene

A phase II trial of arzoxifene, a selective estrogen response modulator, in patients with recurrent or advanced endometrial cancer [55]

Background: Endometrial cancer is hormonally sensitive.

Need to optimize response and minimize toxicity for patients with advanced or recurrent endometrial cancer, many of whom have significant medical co-morbidiites

Arzoxifene is a potent selective estrogen receptor modulator (SERM)

Objective: Determine response rate and toxicity of arzoxifene in patients with recurrent or advanced endometrial cancer

Patients: 37 enrolled; 29 evaluable for efficacy; recurrent or advanced endometrial cancer; estrogen receptor positive (ER+) and/or progesterone receptor positive (PR+) by IHC; measurable disease; patients with serous or clear cell histology excluded

Years: 1999 – 2001

Treatment:

	Arzoxifene 20 mg/day PO (n=29)
Response rate	
Complete response	1 patient
Partial response	8 patients
Stable disease	2 patients
PFS	3.7 months
PFS of CR & PR patients	13.9 months

Conclusions: Arzoxifene demonstrated responses (RR=31%) and longer duration of response in phase II trials to date

Controversies / Questions: ER/PR tested on primary tumor, not recurrent disease

Does response to hormonal therapy vary by site of disease [50, 52]?

Would response be improved if given in combination with tamoxifen via its upregulation of progesterone receptors?

Need for agents with improved response rate as well as duration of response in advanced and recurrent endometrial cancer

Uterine Carcinosarcoma:

Chemotherapy, Radiotherapy in Endometrial Cancer

EORTC 55874

Phase III randomized study to evaluate the role of adjuvant pelvic radiotherapy in the treatment of uterine sarcomas stages I and II: An European Organisation for Research and Treatment of Cancer Gynaecological Cancer Group Study [56]

Background: Reports of post-operative RT improving outcomes in early stage uterine carcinosarcoma (CS)

Objective: To determine if adjuvant pelvic RT reduces the pelvic recurrence rate in patients with surgically resected stage I and II uterine CS

Patients: 224 women with stage I and II CS (n=92), leiomyosarcoma (LMS) (n=99), and endometrial stroma sarcoma (ESS) (n=30) s/p TAH/BSO

Years: 1988 – 2001

Treatment arms:

	Pelvic RT 50.4 Gy (28 fractions)	Observation	P value
PFS	6.22 years	4.93 years	0.3524
OS	8.53 years	6.78 years	0.923
Recurrence (5 yr)			
Local*	18.8%	35.9%	0.0013
Distant	45.3%	33.6%	0.2569

*Better local control with RT for CS, but not for LMS

Conclusions: RT resulted in improved local control for patients with CS, but no survival benefit

No benefit of RT for patients with LMS

Controversies / Questions:

Study included both LMS and CS (two different tumor types)

Improved pelvic control for LMS patients did not translate into survival advantage

What is the role of post-op RT considering its morbidity and inability to impact survival?

GOG108

A Phase III Trial of Ifosfamide with or without Cisplatin in Carcinosarcoma of the Uterus: A Gynecologic Oncology Group Study [57]

Background: Need for effective therapies for uterine carcinosarcoma (CS)

Objective: Determine if addition of cisplatin to ifosfamide improves response rate and survival in patients with uterine CS and to determine the toxicity of the regimen

Patients: 224 enrolled; 194 women eligible with advanced, persistent or recurrent CS of uterus

Years: 1989 - 1996

Treatment arms:

	Ifosfamide* 1.5g/m^2/day IV x 4 days + Mesna	+ cisplatin 20 mg/m^2/day IV x 4 days	P value
	Q 3 wks x 8 cycles		
Median # cycles	4	4	
CR	24%	31%	0.03
PR	12%	23%	
Stable dz.	35%	30%	
PFS	4 months	6 months	0.02

Median survival	7.6 months	9.4 months	0.07
Adverse events			
Leukopenia (≥G3)	58%	87%	<0.05
Thrombocytopenia (≥G3)	5%	58%	<0.05

*Ifosfamide regimen changed to 4 days after toxicity with planned 5 day regimen

Conclusions: The combination of cisplatin + ifosfamide was associated with improvement in response and PFS, but at the expense of significant toxicity, with a short overall survival

Controversies / Questions: Nearly a third of patients discontinued therapy secondary to toxicity or patient refusal (23% in ifosfamide only arm and 43% in ifos + cis arm)

Treatment may have contributed to the death of 6 patients treated with ifos + cis (5 day regimen)

Treatment arms imbalanced with 37% of patients in ifos only arm with measurable disease limited to pelvis vs. 59% in the ifos + cis combo arm

Considering the short increase in PFS and OS, is the added toxicity of the combination arm warranted?

GOG 117

Adjuvant ifosfamide and cisplatin in patients with completely resected stage I or II carcinosarcomas (mixed mesodermal tumors) of the uterus: a Gynecologic Oncology Group study [58]

Background: Early stage carcinosarcomas can recur distally and result in death

Objective: To determine the PFS, OS and toxicity of ifosfamide + cisplatin in patients with completely resected stage I or II CS of uterus

Patients: 65 evaluable patients with stage I (77%) and II (23%) carcinosarcoma of uterus s/p TAH/BSO

Years: 1991 – 1993

Treatment:

	Ifosfamide 1.5 g/m^2 IV x 4 days* (with Mesna) Cisplatin 20 mg/m^2 IV x 4 days* Q 3 weeks x 3
PFS (24 months)	69%
OS (24 months)	82%
OS (5 year)	62%
Adverse events	
Thrombocytopenia (≥G3)	63%

| Neutropenia (≥G3) | 26% |

*4 day regimen is result of dose reduction of originally planned 5 day regimen secondary to myelotoxicity

Conclusions: Adjuvant ifosfamide + cisplatin for patients with stage I and II CS is tolerable, however with no controls difficult to assess the input of ifos+cisplatin on PFS and OS

Controversies / Questions: Half of recurrences involved the pelvis. Would adjuvant pelvic RT be beneficial in decreasing this risk?

LND not required for study enrollment. How many patients had occult metastatic disease?

Patients were treated with only 3 cycles of chemotherapy

Follow-up: In a multi-institutional study by Cantrell et al [59], for women with FIGO stage I-II uterine carcinosarcoma, PFS was improved with adjuvant chemotherapy versus radiation or observation alone. Chemotherapy regimens included: cisplatin + ifosfamide and paclitaxel + carboplatin

GOG 150

A gynecologic oncology group randomized phase III trial of whole abdominal irradiation (WAI) vs. cisplatin-ifosfamide and mesna (CIM) as post-surgical therapy in stage I–IV carcinosarcoma (CS) of the uterus [60]

Background: Uterine CS's have a propensity to recur, often in the pelvis, which has been shown to be decreased with RT [61]

GOG 117 demonstrated the feasibility of ifosfamide + cisplatin

Objective: Compare whole abdominal irradiation (WAI) versus ifosfamide + cisplatin with respect to OS, recurrence and toxicity in patients with uterine CS

Patients: 206 women with stage I, II, III, and IV primary CS of uterus or cervix (without liver parenchymal or extra-abdominal disease) s/p TAH, BSO, cytoreduction to <1cm (stage III (disease outside uterus but not outside pelvis) most common (45%))

Years: 1993 – 2005

Treatment arms:

	WAI* EBRT to abdomen (30Gy) + pelvic boost (20 Gy)	**cisplatin** 20mg/m^2/day x 4 days Q 3 weeks x 3 cycles + **ifosfamide** 1.5 g/m^2/day x 4 days (with Mesna)	P value
Recurrence (5 yr) ∞	**58%**	**52%**	0.245
Recurrence (5 yr)	21% lower with ifos + cisplatin‡		
Survival (5 yr)	35%	45%	0.085
Survival (5 yr)	29% lower with ifos + cisplatin		
Toxicity			
Anemia (≥G3)	1%	11%	<0.01
Chronic GI(≥G2)	10%	0%	<0.001
Neuropathy (≥G3)	0%	9%	

*borders: superior: diaphragm; inferior: inguinal ligaments; lateral: peritoneal margin

‡ adjusted for stage of disease and age at diagnosis

∞ There is a discrepancy in the published paper regarding the % reduction in recurrence rate in the abstract (21%) and the results section (29%)

Conclusions: No difference in relapse rate or OS between ifosfamide + cisplatin versus WAI; "CIM appeared to have a slight advantage and was not more toxic."

Controversies / Questions: Completion of a large clinical trial for this rare tumor type is difficult. Took 12 years to enroll 232 patients.

Only 3 cycles administered (vs. GOG 108 and GOG 161). Were patients undertreated?

Recurrence rate higher for Black women versus White women

Pattern of pelvic and distant recurrences similar between groups, but vaginal recurrences were increased in chemo arm (10 vs. 4) and abdomen recurrences decreased in chemo arm (19 vs. 29).

Is there a role for vaginal brachytherapy combined with chemotherapy?

GOG 161

Phase III Trial of Ifosfamide With or Without Paclitaxel in Advanced Uterine Carcinosarcoma: A Gynecologic Oncology Group Study [62]

Background: Ifosfamide + cisplatin demonstrated superior response rates versus ifosfamide alone, but no survival advantage, for patients with uterine CS [57]

Paclitaxel with activity in CS [63]

Objective: Determine if addition of paclitaxel to ifosfamide improves PFS, OS, response for patients with advanced uterine CS

Patients: 179 women with stage III or IV, persistent or recurrent uterine CS

Years: 1997 – 2004

Treatment arms:

	Ifosfamide 2 gm/m^2 IV x 3 days (+Mesna)	**Ifosfamide** 1.6 gm/m^2 IV x 3 days (+Mesna) + **Paclitaxel** 135 mg/m^2	P value
	Q 21 days x up to 8 cycles		
Response rate	29%	45%	0.02*
PFS	3.6 months	5.8 months	0.03*
OS	8.4 months	13.5 months	0.03*
Adverse events			

| Periph neuropathy(G1-4) | 8% | 30% | <0.05 |
| Neutropenia (≥G3) | 53% | 44% | >0.05 |

*stratified by performance status

Conclusions: OS was significantly improved with combination of ifosfamide + paclitaxel, however new active agents are needed considering the poor OS

Controversies / Questions: More patients with measurable disease confined to pelvis in the ifos + paclitaxel arm vs. ifos alone arm (37% vs. 23%), but more patients with pelvic + extrapelvic disease (29%) in ifosfamide only arm versus ifos + paclitaxel arm (19%)

Ifosfamide as single agent dosed higher than ifos in combination arm

No QOL assessment

How did a 2 month improvement in PFS translate to a 5 month improvement in OS?

Leiomyosarcoma (LMS):

Chemotherapy, Radiotherapy in Uterine LMS

GOG 131C

Evaluation of paclitaxel in previously treated leiomyosarcoma of the uterus: a gynecologic oncology group study [64]

Background: A need to identify active chemotherapy in advanced and recurrent LMS

Objective: Evaluate the efficacy of paclitaxel in patients with recurrent or advanced uterine LMS

Patients: 48 patients with LMS with measurable disease; ≤1 prior non-paclitaxel chemotherapy regimen

Years: 1997 – 2000

Treatment:

	Paclitaxel 175 mg/m^2 IV (if no prior RT) or **Paclitaxel** 135 mg/m^2 IV (if prior RT)
	Q 3 weeks
Median number of cycles	2
Complete response	4.2%*
Partial response	4.2%
Stable dz.	22.9%
PFS	1.5 months (range: 0.5 – 22.2 months)
OS	12.1 months (range: 1.2 – 39.3 months

Adverse events	
Neutropenia (≥G3)	16.7%
Anemia (≥G3)	16.7%

*2 patients (1 with disease in lung only and 1 with disease in liver only)

Conclusions: Paclitaxel demonstrated "modest" activity in patients with previously treated advanced or recurrent LMS

GOG 131E

Phase II trial of gemcitabine as second-line chemotherapy of uterine leiomyosarcoma: a Gynecologic Oncology Group (GOG) Study [65]

Background: Majority of patients with recurrent uterine LMS may be candidates for systemic cytotoxic therapy, but without evidence of cure. Need to search for chemotherapies with a more durable response.

Objective: To assess the response rate and toxicity of gemcitabine in patients with persistent, recurrent, unresectable uterine LMS

Patients: 44 patients with recurrent or persistent LMS (majority with prior cytotoxic therapy)

Years: 1998 – 2001

Treatment:

	Gemcitabine 1,000 mg/m^2 IV over 30 min. Days 1, 8, 15 (Q28 days)
Response rate (CR + PR)	20.5%
Complete Response	2.3%
Partial Response	18.2%
Stable disease	15.9%
Duration of response (median)	4.9 months

Adverse events	
Neutropenia (≥G3)	34%
Thrombocytopenia (≥G3)	11%

Conclusions: Gemcitabine demonstrates activity, with a favorable toxicity profile, in patients with persistent or recurrent uterine LMS and should be considered in multiagent regimens.

Controversies / Questions: Would a longer gemcitabine infusion allow for more sustained DNA synthesis inhibitory concentrations and improved efficacy?

Which chemotherapy should gemcitabine be paired with in a combination chemotherapy regimen?

Hensley (unresectable LMS)

Gemcitabine and Docetaxel in Patients With Unresectable Leiomyosarcoma: Results of a Phase II Trial [66]

<u>Background</u>: Treatment options for advanced, recurrent LMS are limited

<u>Objective</u>: Determine the clinical activity of docetaxel + gemcitabine in unresectable LMS

<u>Patients</u>: 34 patients with LMS; majority (85%) uterine origin

<u>Years</u>: Not listed

<u>Treatment</u>:

	Gemcitabine 900 mg/m² Days #1, 8 **Docetaxel** 100 mg/m² Day #8 Q 3 weeks x 6 cycles
Response rate (CR + PR)	53%
Complete response	9%
Partial response	44%
Stable dz	21%
PFS	5.6 months
OS	17.9 months
Adverse events	
Neutropenia (≥G3)	21%
Thrombocytopenia (≥G3)	29%
Anemia (≥G3)	15%

Conclusions: Gemcitabine + docetaxel is active in LMS

Controversies: The favorable response rates should be confirmed in a larger multi-institutional trial

Hensley (resectable LMS)

Adjuvant gemcitabine plus docetaxel for completely resected stages I-IV high grade uterine leiomyosarcoma: Results of a prospective study [67]

Background: Early stage LMS has high risk of recurrence

Gemcitabine + docetaxel with activity in advanced, recurrent uterine LMS

Objective: Determine whether adjuvant gemcitabine + docetaxel improves PFS in patients with completely resected stage I – IV uterine LMS

Patients: 23 patients with uterine LMS (15 with stage I) s/p TAH (at least)

Years: 2002 – 2006

Treatment:

	Gemcitabine 900 mg/m^2 Days #1, 8 & **Docetaxel** 75 mg/m^2 Day #1
	Q 3 weeks x 4
PFS	13 months
PFS (stage I and II)	39 months*
OS (stage I and II)	>49 months‡

*59% progression free at 2 years ‡Not yet reached

Conclusions: Gemcitabine + docetaxel yields improved PFS (compared to historical controls)

Controversies / Questions: Small, single institution study

Comparison group = historical controls

GOG 131G

Fixed-dose rate gemcitabine plus docetaxel as first-line therapy for metastatic uterine leiomyosarcoma: A Gynecologic Oncology Group phase II trial [68]

Background: Gemcitabine + docetaxel has demonstrated activity as 2nd line therapy for metastatic uterine leiomyosarcoma (LMS) [66]

Objective: Determine the activity of gemcitabine + docetaxel in women with advanced LMS

Patients: 42 patients with advanced, unresectable LMS; measurable disease; no prior cytotoxic therapy

Years: 2003 - 2006

Treatment:

	Gemcitabine 900 mg/m^2 IV over 90 minutes Days #1, 8 & **Docetaxel** 100 mg/m^2 IV over 1 hour Day #8
	Q 3 weeks
Response rate (CR + PR)	36%
Complete response	5%
Partial response	31%
Stable dz	26%

PFS	4.4 months (range: 0.4 – 37$^+$ months)
OS	16.1 months (range: 0.4 – 31.3 months)
Adverse effects	
Neutropenia (≥G3)	17%
Anemia (≥G3)	24%
Thrombocytopenia (≥G3)	14%

Conclusions: Gemcitabine + docetaxel is a reasonable option for first line treatment of metastatic uterine LMS

Controversies / Questions: The duration of responses is quite varied among patients

GOG 87J

Phase II evaluation of liposomal doxorubicin (Doxil) in recurrent or advanced leiomyosarcoma of the uterus: a Gynecologic oncology Group study [69]

Background: Patients with metastatic LMS have a poor prognosis

Objective: Evaluate clinical response and toxicity of liposomal doxorubicin (Doxil) in patients with advanced or recurrent LMS

Patients: 31 patients with advanced or recurrent LMS considered incurable; chemotherapy naive

Years: 2000 – 2001

Treatment:

	Doxil 50 mg/m^2 IV Q 4 weeks
Median number of cycles	2
Complete response	3%
Partial response	13%
Stable disease	32%
Duration of response	4.1 months (range: 1.6 – 6 months)
Adverse events	
Neutropenia (≥G3)	16%
PPE (≥G3)	6.5%
Anemia (≥G3)	23%

Conclusions: The dose and schedule of Doxil used in this trial showed no advantage over doxorubicin [70, 71]

Impact: "further evaluation of single agent liposomal doxorubicin in this patient population does not seem warranted"

Controversies / Questions: While cross-trial comparisons have limitations, compare these results with those of Hensley et al [66] evaluating the efficacy of docetaxel + gemcitabine in patients with unresectable LMS, including 47% who had previously received doxorubicin with or without ifosfamide

Special Topics

KEYNOTE-028

Safety and Antitumor Activity of Pembrolizumab in Advanced Programmed Death Ligand 1-Positive Endometrial Cancer: Results from the KEYNOTE-028 Study [72]

Background: Treatment options for those with advanced and recurrent endometrial cancer are limited

Objective: Evaluate the safety and efficacy of pembrolizumab, an anti-programmed death 1 monoclonal antibody, in patients with PD-L1(+) endometrial cancer

Patients: 24 patients with PD-L1 (+) endometrial cancer from the KEYNOTE-028 trial

Treatment:

	Pembrolizumab 10 mg/kg IV Q 2 weeks (max of 24 months or until disease progression)
Complete response	0%
Partial response	13%*
Stable disease	13%‡
Adverse events	
Fatigue	21%
Pruritis	17%
Pyrexia	13%
Decreased appetite	13%

*median duration not reached; duration of response for these 3 pts: 64+, 65+, & 64 wks

‡median duration of stable disease 24.6 weeks

Conclusions: Pembrolizumab shows promise as a treatment for advanced endometrial cancer with a favorable safety profile and durable responses

Controversies / Questions:

What % of patients with advanced or recurrent endometrial cancer are PD-L1 (+)?

Will pembrolizumab be more effective in patients with POLE mutations?

What is the role of pembrolizumab in combination with other therapies?

GOG 137

Randomized Double-Blind Trial of Estrogen Replacement Therapy Versus Placebo in Stage I or II Endometrial Cancer: A Gynecologic Oncology Group Study [73]

Background: Adenocarcinoma of the endometrium is an estrogen-dependent cancer.

Concern that estrogen use could stimulate occult disease.

Objective: Determine the effect of estrogen replacement therapy in women with a history of stage I or II endometrial cancer

Patients: 1,236 women with stage I or II endometrial adenocarcinoma treated with hyst + BSO +/- LND with indication for estrogen replacement therapy (ERT)

Years: 1997 – 2003

Treatment:

		Placebo	ERT
		Stage I or II endometrial adenocarcinoma (any grade) s/p hyst, BSO +/- LND	
Median age		57 years	
Stage			
	IA	39%	38%
	IB	49%	50%
	IC	7%	8%

	II	5%	5%
Median follow-up		36 months	
Recurrences		1.9%	2.3%
Death from endometrial cancer		0.6%	0.8%

Conclusions: Absolute risk of recurrence low, although study unable to conclusively refute or support the safety of exogenous estrogen.

Controversies / Questions: Study closed prematurely (secondary to abundance of patients with early, good prognosis tumors and poor accrual after announcement that the estrogen + progestin arm of the WHI was being stopped) and therefore not able to answer question trial was designed for.

Majority of patients at low risk for recurrence.

Of patients taking placebo, 38% believed they were on ERT arm.

References

1. Siegel, R.L., K.D. Miller, and A. Jemal, *Cancer statistics, 2016.* CA Cancer J Clin, 2016. **66**(1): p. 7-30.

2. Zaino, R.J., et al., *Reproducibility of the diagnosis of atypical endometrial hyperplasia: a Gynecologic Oncology Group study.* Cancer, 2006. **106**(4): p. 804-11.

3. Kurman, R.J., P.F. Kaminski, and H.J. Norris, *The behavior of endometrial hyperplasia. A long-term study of "untreated" hyperplasia in 170 patients.* Cancer, 1985. **56**(2): p. 403-12.

4. Allison, K.H., et al., *Diagnosing endometrial hyperplasia: why is it so difficult to agree?* Am J Surg Pathol, 2008. **32**(5): p. 691-8.

5. Lax, S.F., et al., *A binary architectural grading system for uterine endometrial endometrioid carcinoma has superior reproducibility compared with FIGO grading and identifies subsets of advance-stage tumors with favorable and unfavorable prognosis.* Am J Surg Pathol, 2000. **24**(9): p. 1201-8.

6. Scholten, A.N., et al., *Prognostic significance and interobserver variability of histologic grading systems for endometrial carcinoma.* Cancer, 2004. **100**(4): p. 764-72.

7. Trimble, C.L., et al., *Concurrent endometrial carcinoma in women with a biopsy diagnosis of atypical*

endometrial hyperplasia: a Gynecologic Oncology Group study. Cancer, 2006. **106**(4): p. 812-9.

8. Trimble, C.L., et al., *Management of endometrial precancers.* Obstet Gynecol, 2012. **120**(5): p. 1160-75.

9. Creasman, W.T., et al., *Surgical pathologic spread patterns of endometrial cancer. A Gynecologic Oncology Group Study.* Cancer, 1987. **60**(8 Suppl): p. 2035-41.

10. Walker, J.L., et al., *Laparoscopy compared with laparotomy for comprehensive surgical staging of uterine cancer: Gynecologic Oncology Group Study LAP2.* J Clin Oncol, 2009. **27**(32): p. 5331-6.

11. Vergote, I., F. Amant, and P. Neven, *Is it safe to treat endometrial carcinoma endoscopically?* J Clin Oncol, 2009. **27**(32): p. 5305-7.

12. Galaal, K., et al., *Laparoscopy versus laparotomy for the management of early stage endometrial cancer.* Cochrane Database Syst Rev, 2012. **9**: p. CD006655.

13. Janda, M., et al., *Effect of Total Laparoscopic Hysterectomy vs Total Abdominal Hysterectomy on Disease-Free Survival Among Women With Stage I Endometrial Cancer: A Randomized Clinical Trial.* JAMA, 2017. **317**(12): p. 1224-1233.

14. group, A.s., et al., *Efficacy of systematic pelvic lymphadenectomy in endometrial cancer (MRC ASTEC trial): a randomised study.* Lancet, 2009. **373**(9658): p. 125-36.

15. Amant, F., P. Neven, and I. Vergote, *Lymphadenectomy in endometrial cancer.* Lancet, 2009. **373**(9670): p. 1169-70; author reply 1170-1.

16. Hakmi, A., *Lymphadenectomy in endometrial cancer.* Lancet, 2009. **373**(9670): p. 1169; author reply 1170-1.

17. Hockel, M. and N. Dornhofer, *Treatment of early endometrial carcinoma: is less more?* Lancet, 2009. **373**(9658): p. 97-9.

18. Mourits, M.J., C.B. Bijen, and G.H. de Bock, *Lymphadenectomy in endometrial cancer.* Lancet, 2009. **373**(9670): p. 1169; author reply 1170-1.

19. Uccella, S., et al., *Lymphadenectomy in endometrial cancer.* Lancet, 2009. **373**(9670): p. 1170; author reply 1170-1.

20. Creasman, W.T., D.E. Mutch, and T.J. Herzog, *ASTEC lymphadenectomy and radiation therapy studies: are conclusions valid?* Gynecol Oncol, 2010. **116**(3): p. 293-4.

21. Benedetti Panici, P., et al., *Systematic pelvic lymphadenectomy vs. no lymphadenectomy in early-stage endometrial carcinoma: randomized clinical trial.* J Natl Cancer Inst, 2008. **100**(23): p. 1707-16.

22. Bristow, R.E., et al., *FIGO stage IIIC endometrial carcinoma: resection of macroscopic nodal disease and other determinants of survival.* Int J Gynecol Cancer, 2003. **13**(5): p. 664-72.

23. Seamon, L.G., J.M. Fowler, and D.E. Cohn, *Lymphadenectomy for endometrial cancer: the controversy.* Gynecol Oncol, 2010. **117**(1): p. 6-8.

24. Walsh, C.S. and B.Y. Karlan, *Lymphadenectomy's role in early endometrial cancer: prognostic or therapeutic?* J Natl Cancer Inst, 2008. **100**(23): p. 1660-1.

25. Keys, H.M., et al., *A phase III trial of surgery with or without adjunctive external pelvic radiation therapy in intermediate risk endometrial adenocarcinoma: a Gynecologic Oncology Group study.* Gynecol Oncol, 2004. **92**(3): p. 744-51.

26. Berman, M.L., *Adjuvant radiotherapy following properly staged endometrial cancer: what role?* Gynecol Oncol, 2004. **92**(3): p. 737-9.

27. Creutzberg, C.L., *GOG-99: ending the controversy regarding pelvic radiotherapy for endometrial carcinoma?* Gynecol Oncol, 2004. **92**(3): p. 740-3.

28. Creutzberg, C.L., et al., *Surgery and postoperative radiotherapy versus surgery alone for patients with stage-1 endometrial carcinoma: multicentre randomised trial. PORTEC Study Group. Post Operative Radiation Therapy in Endometrial Carcinoma.* Lancet, 2000. **355**(9213): p. 1404-11.

29. Burger, M.P. and B.W. Mol, *Treatment for patients with stage-1 endometrial carcinoma.* Lancet, 2000. **356**(9232): p. 853-4.

30. Look, K.Y., *Who benefits from radiotherapy in treatment of endometrial cancer and at what price?* Lancet, 2000. **355**(9213): p. 1381-2.

31. Nout, R.A., et al., *Vaginal brachytherapy versus pelvic external beam radiotherapy for patients with endometrial cancer of high-intermediate risk (PORTEC-2): an open-label, non-inferiority, randomised trial.* Lancet, 2010. **375**(9717): p. 816-23.

32. Kitchener, H. and M. Powell, *Radiotherapy for endometrial cancer: a key piece in the jigsaw.* Lancet, 2010. **375**(9717): p. 781-2.

33. Nout, R.A., et al., *Quality of life after pelvic radiotherapy or vaginal brachytherapy for endometrial cancer: first results of the randomized PORTEC-2 trial.* J Clin Oncol, 2009. **27**(21): p. 3547-56.

34. Maggi, R., et al., *Adjuvant chemotherapy vs radiotherapy in high-risk endometrial carcinoma: results of a randomised trial.* Br J Cancer, 2006. **95**(3): p. 266-71.

35. Susumu, N., et al., *Randomized phase III trial of pelvic radiotherapy versus cisplatin-based combined chemotherapy in patients with intermediate- and high-risk endometrial cancer: a Japanese Gynecologic Oncology Group study.* Gynecol Oncol, 2008. **108**(1): p. 226-33.

36. Thigpen, J.T., et al., *A randomized comparison of doxorubicin alone versus doxorubicin plus cyclophosphamide in the management of advanced or recurrent endometrial carcinoma: A Gynecologic*

Oncology Group study. *J Clin Oncol*, 1994. **12**(7): p. 1408-14.

37. Thigpen, J.T., et al., *Phase III trial of doxorubicin with or without cisplatin in advanced endometrial carcinoma: a gynecologic oncology group study.* J Clin Oncol, 2004. **22**(19): p. 3902-8.

38. Fleming, G.F., et al., *Phase III randomized trial of doxorubicin + cisplatin versus doxorubicin + 24-h paclitaxel + filgrastim in endometrial carcinoma: a Gynecologic Oncology Group study.* Ann Oncol, 2004. **15**(8): p. 1173-8.

39. Gallion, H.H., et al., *Randomized phase III trial of standard timed doxorubicin plus cisplatin versus circadian timed doxorubicin plus cisplatin in stage III and IV or recurrent endometrial carcinoma: a Gynecologic Oncology Group Study.* J Clin Oncol, 2003. **21**(20): p. 3808-13.

40. Fleming, G.F., et al., *Phase III trial of doxorubicin plus cisplatin with or without paclitaxel plus filgrastim in advanced endometrial carcinoma: a Gynecologic Oncology Group Study.* J Clin Oncol, 2004. **22**(11): p. 2159-66.

41. McMeekin, D.S., et al., *The relationship between histology and outcome in advanced and recurrent endometrial cancer patients participating in first-line chemotherapy trials: a Gynecologic Oncology Group study.* Gynecol Oncol, 2007. **106**(1): p. 16-22.

42. Muggia, F.M., et al., *Phase II trial of the pegylated liposomal doxorubicin in previously treated metastatic*

endometrial cancer: a Gynecologic Oncology Group study. J Clin Oncol, 2002. **20**(9): p. 2360-4.

43. Fleming, G.F., et al., *Phase II trial of trastuzumab in women with advanced or recurrent, HER2-positive endometrial carcinoma: a Gynecologic Oncology Group study.* Gynecol Oncol, 2010. **116**(1): p. 15-20.

44. Aghajanian, C., et al., *Phase II trial of bevacizumab in recurrent or persistent endometrial cancer: a Gynecologic Oncology Group study.* J Clin Oncol, 2011. **29**(16): p. 2259-65.

45. Randall, M.E., et al., *Randomized phase III trial of whole-abdominal irradiation versus doxorubicin and cisplatin chemotherapy in advanced endometrial carcinoma: a Gynecologic Oncology Group Study.* J Clin Oncol, 2006. **24**(1): p. 36-44.

46. Smith, R.S., et al., *Treatment of high-risk uterine cancer with whole abdominopelvic radiation therapy.* Int J Radiat Oncol Biol Phys, 2000. **48**(3): p. 767-78.

47. Homesley, H.D., et al., *A randomized phase III trial in advanced endometrial carcinoma of surgery and volume directed radiation followed by cisplatin and doxorubicin with or without paclitaxel: A Gynecologic Oncology Group study.* Gynecol Oncol, 2009. **112**(3): p. 543-52.

48. Thigpen, J.T., et al., *Oral medroxyprogesterone acetate in the treatment of advanced or recurrent endometrial carcinoma: a dose-response study by the Gynecologic Oncology Group.* J Clin Oncol, 1999. **17**(6): p. 1736-44.

49. Thigpen, T., et al., *Tamoxifen in the treatment of advanced or recurrent endometrial carcinoma: a Gynecologic Oncology Group study.* J Clin Oncol, 2001. **19**(2): p. 364-7.

50. Lentz, S.S., et al., *High-dose megestrol acetate in advanced or recurrent endometrial carcinoma: a Gynecologic Oncology Group Study.* J Clin Oncol, 1996. **14**(2): p. 357-61.

51. Whitney, C.W., et al., *Phase II study of medroxyprogesterone acetate plus tamoxifen in advanced endometrial carcinoma: a Gynecologic Oncology Group study.* Gynecol Oncol, 2004. **92**(1): p. 4-9.

52. Fiorica, J.V., et al., *Phase II trial of alternating courses of megestrol acetate and tamoxifen in advanced endometrial carcinoma: a Gynecologic Oncology Group study.* Gynecol Oncol, 2004. **92**(1): p. 10-4.

53. Rose, P.G., et al., *A phase II trial of anastrozole in advanced recurrent or persistent endometrial carcinoma: a Gynecologic Oncology Group study.* Gynecol Oncol, 2000. **78**(2): p. 212-6.

54. Kauppila, A., *Progestin therapy of endometrial, breast and ovarian carcinoma. A review of clinical observations.* Acta Obstet Gynecol Scand, 1984. **63**(5): p. 441-50.

55. McMeekin, D.S., et al., *A phase II trial of arzoxifene, a selective estrogen response modulator, in patients with recurrent or advanced endometrial cancer.* Gynecol Oncol, 2003. **90**(1): p. 64-9.

56. Reed, N.S., et al., *Phase III randomised study to evaluate the role of adjuvant pelvic radiotherapy in the treatment of uterine sarcomas stages I and II: an European Organisation for Research and Treatment of Cancer Gynaecological Cancer Group Study (protocol 55874).* Eur J Cancer, 2008. **44**(6): p. 808-18.

57. Sutton, G., et al., *A phase III trial of ifosfamide with or without cisplatin in carcinosarcoma of the uterus: A Gynecologic Oncology Group Study.* Gynecol Oncol, 2000. **79**(2): p. 147-53.

58. Sutton, G., et al., *Adjuvant ifosfamide and cisplatin in patients with completely resected stage I or II carcinosarcomas (mixed mesodermal tumors) of the uterus: a Gynecologic Oncology Group study.* Gynecol Oncol, 2005. **96**(3): p. 630-4.

59. Cantrell, L.A., et al., *A multi-institutional cohort study of adjuvant therapy in stage I-II uterine carcinosarcoma.* Gynecol Oncol, 2012. **127**(1): p. 22-6.

60. Wolfson, A.H., et al., *A gynecologic oncology group randomized phase III trial of whole abdominal irradiation (WAI) vs. cisplatin-ifosfamide and mesna (CIM) as post-surgical therapy in stage I-IV carcinosarcoma (CS) of the uterus.* Gynecol Oncol, 2007. **107**(2): p. 177-85.

61. Hornback, N.B., G. Omura, and F.J. Major, *Observations on the use of adjuvant radiation therapy in patients with stage I and II uterine sarcoma.* Int J Radiat Oncol Biol Phys, 1986. **12**(12): p. 2127-30.

62. Homesley, H.D., et al., *Phase III trial of ifosfamide with or without paclitaxel in advanced uterine carcinosarcoma: a Gynecologic Oncology Group Study.* J Clin Oncol, 2007. **25**(5): p. 526-31.

63. Curtin, J.P., et al., *Paclitaxel in the treatment of carcinosarcoma of the uterus: a gynecologic oncology group study.* Gynecol Oncol, 2001. **83**(2): p. 268-70.

64. Gallup, D.G., et al., *Evaluation of paclitaxel in previously treated leiomyosarcoma of the uterus: a gynecologic oncology group study.* Gynecol Oncol, 2003. **89**(1): p. 48-51.

65. Look, K.Y., et al., *Phase II trial of gemcitabine as second-line chemotherapy of uterine leiomyosarcoma: a Gynecologic Oncology Group (GOG) Study.* Gynecol Oncol, 2004. **92**(2): p. 644-7.

66. Hensley, M.L., et al., *Gemcitabine and docetaxel in patients with unresectable leiomyosarcoma: results of a phase II trial.* J Clin Oncol, 2002. **20**(12): p. 2824-31.

67. Hensley, M.L., et al., *Adjuvant gemcitabine plus docetaxel for completely resected stages I-IV high grade uterine leiomyosarcoma: Results of a prospective study.* Gynecol Oncol, 2009. **112**(3): p. 563-7.

68. Hensley, M.L., et al., *Fixed-dose rate gemcitabine plus docetaxel as first-line therapy for metastatic uterine leiomyosarcoma: a Gynecologic Oncology Group phase II trial.* Gynecol Oncol, 2008. **109**(3): p. 329-34.

69. Sutton, G., et al., *Phase II evaluation of liposomal doxorubicin (Doxil) in recurrent or advanced leiomyosarcoma of the uterus: a Gynecologic Oncology Group study.* Gynecol Oncol, 2005. **96**(3): p. 749-52.

70. Muss, H.B., et al., *Treatment of recurrent or advanced uterine sarcoma. A randomized trial of doxorubicin versus doxorubicin and cyclophosphamide (a phase III trial of the Gynecologic Oncology Group).* Cancer, 1985. **55**(8): p. 1648-53.

71. Omura, G.A., et al., *A randomized study of adriamycin with and without dimethyl triazenoimidazole carboxamide in advanced uterine sarcomas.* Cancer, 1983. **52**(4): p. 626-32.

72. Ott, P.A., et al., *Safety and Antitumor Activity of Pembrolizumab in Advanced Programmed Death Ligand 1-Positive Endometrial Cancer: Results From the KEYNOTE-028 Study.* J Clin Oncol, 2017. **35**(22): p. 2535-2541.

73. Barakat, R.R., et al., *Randomized double-blind trial of estrogen replacement therapy versus placebo in stage I or II endometrial cancer: a Gynecologic Oncology Group Study.* J Clin Oncol, 2006. **24**(4): p. 587-92.

Made in the USA
Middletown, DE
26 June 2019